DEFEATING DOWN SYNDROME WITH EXPERT GUIDANCE

Ultimate Solution Handbook For Patients, Guardians Or Family To Understand, Manage, Treat, Prevent, Reverse Symptoms And Live Well

DR. POTTER WHITLEY

approval or validation is not implied by the inclusion of these references.

Any direct, indirect, incidental, special, or consequential damages resulting from using or not being able to use the material in this book are not covered by the author's liability policy. For medical advice and counsel particular to their circumstances, readers are advised to check with experienced healthcare specialists.

The content, materials, and information in this book are subject to change at any time without prior notice, at the author's discretion. The text may contain errors or omissions for which the author is not responsible.

By reading this book, you understand and accept the conditions of this disclaimer.

THE REASON BEHIND THIS BOOK

For those navigating the complicated world of Down syndrome, "Defeating Down Syndrome with Expert Guidance" is an invaluable resource for professionals, families, and people. This book delves into the intricacies of comprehending Down syndrome, emphasizing the vital requirement for expert aid. By providing a comprehensive overview that makes clear the genetic basis, causes, and range of severity associated with the condition, it advances a deeper understanding of Down syndrome.

One of the key benefits of this book is its emphasis on early diagnosis and intervention. It covers prenatal testing, counseling, and early symptom recognition to highlight the critical importance of timely intervention programs. With viewpoints from genetic counselors, pediatricians, and specialty therapists, the narrative skillfully transitions into the critical function of professional assessment and help, offering a thorough approach to care.

Thoroughly thought-out teaching strategies are discussed, with a focus on the need to develop individualized lesson plans, implement inclusive education models, and leverage instructional technology that has been modified to meet the unique needs of individuals with Down syndrome. In addition to discussing medical issues and regular checkups, this book also discusses the importance of wellness and nutrition, as well as common health issues that are specific to those with Down syndrome.

The narrative takes a more compassionate approach to psychosocial development, emphasizing the value of social skills and emotional intelligence development as well as the crucial role that family and community support play in the lives of individuals with Down syndrome. The treatment modalities—physical therapy, occupational therapy, and speech and language therapy—that have been discussed provide a way ahead for enhancing the overall well-being and standard of living of individuals with Down syndrome.

This article explores the ground-breaking findings and ongoing investigations into Down syndrome, offering a synopsis of recent advancements, workable therapies, and possible directions for future research. By giving parents the knowledge and resources they need to defend the rights and welfare of their children, this book puts parents in control.

An inspiring final section of the narrative showcases the successes and accomplishments of individuals with Down syndrome. By embracing diversity and dispelling stereotypes, this book encourages readers to feel empowered and uplifted, so bolstering the notion that everyone can have a successful and fulfilling life, regardless of their skill level.

TABLE OF CONTENT

CHAPTER ONE

INTRODUCTION

The etiology of Down syndrome is a genetic duplicate of chromosome 21. This disorder, also known as trisomy 21, results in intellectual and developmental disabilities, distinct physical characteristics, and potential health issues. Professional help is crucial for the care and support of individuals with Down syndrome, even if there is currently no known treatment for the condition. This in-depth analysis delves into the nuances of Down syndrome, shedding light on its complexity and emphasizing the need for expert support to enhance the quality of life for individuals affected.

Understanding Down syndrome:

Investigating the genetic underpinnings of Down syndrome is necessary to comprehend the disorder. In a human, each cell contains 46 chromosomes, which are arranged in 23 pairs. Down syndrome is caused by an extra copy of chromosome 21, which can be the result of a cell division error that occurs early in the embryo's development or during the generation of reproductive cells. The additional genetic material disrupts the typical developmental trajectory, resulting in the development of features unique to Down syndrome.

People with Down syndrome frequently have physical traits like protruding tongues, flat nasal bridges, and almond-shaped eyes. Apart from these apparent signs and symptoms, intellectual deficits and developmental delays have also been linked to the condition. Since each person's experience with these challenges can vary widely, expert supervision is required to tailor therapies to each patient's unique needs.

Individuals with Down syndrome may be more vulnerable to certain health issues such as thyroid problems, respiratory illnesses, and cardiac abnormalities in addition to developmental and cognitive traits. Schools, families, and healthcare providers must be aware of these potential challenges to provide complete care and support. To address the diverse needs of individuals with Down syndrome, a multidisciplinary approach involving educators, therapists, and medical professionals is typically recommended.

Importance of Professional Counsel

Expert assistance is necessary to navigate the challenges associated with Down syndrome. To give individualized interventions, educators, support networks, and healthcare practitioners are working together in this collaborative effort. It is particularly crucial to intervene early since it can significantly affect how people with Down syndrome develop.

Among the several medical professionals who are crucial for correctly diagnosing patients, informing families about possible health issues, and helping them with medical treatment strategies are pediatricians and genetic counselors. Early therapies that improve cognitive and motor skills, such as physical, occupational, and speech therapy, can help people with Down syndrome become more independent.

The knowledge and skills of educational professionals, like learning specialists and special education teachers, are invaluable in fostering inclusive and supportive learning environments. By customizing teaching methods to the unique learning styles and capacities of individuals with Down syndrome, social integration, and academic success can be encouraged. Professional guidance also includes family support and community service to offer a broad network of support that extends beyond the individual.

In conclusion, conquering the challenges presented by Down syndrome requires collaboration, a complete understanding of the condition, and the invaluable counsel of professionals. To help society establish inclusive and supportive environments that enable people with Down syndrome to live happy, productive lives, it is important to understand the hereditary roots of the condition and the importance of professional assistance.

CHAPTER TWO

A BRIEF OVERVIEW OF DOWN SYNDROME
Genetic Basis and Contributing Factors

Down syndrome is a genetic disease characterized by an extra copy of chromosome 21. This condition, also known as trisomy 21, arises in the early stages of fetal development or when reproductive cells are developing. The non-inherited form of Down syndrome, which results from a random error in cell division, accounts for about 95% of cases. Maternal age is a significant factor, as it increases the likelihood of having a child with Down syndrome.

In addition to non-inherited trisomy 21, two less common genetic defects that can produce Down syndrome are mosaicism and translocation. Individuals with mosaicism have different cell types;

some have 46 chromosomes, while others have an extra copy of chromosome 21. Part of chromosome 21 is joined to another chromosome, commonly chromosome 14, in a translocation. In this case, the extra genetic material may still lead to Down syndrome even though there are still 46 chromosomes overall.

Understanding the underlying genetic causes of Down syndrome is crucial to developing preventative and therapeutic strategies. Prenatal diagnostics, such as amniocentesis or chorionic villus sampling (CVS), can help identify the illness early in pregnancy and provide parents with the knowledge they need to make decisions about their child's medical care.

Characteristics of the Mind and Body

Individuals with Down syndrome have a distinct set of physical and cognitive characteristics that vary widely amongst themselves. A short neck, a flat facial profile, and almond-shaped eyes are examples of physical traits. Furthermore, individuals with Down syndrome frequently have a single crease across the palm of their hands and a noticeable separation between their first and second toes. It is often possible to identify these physical characteristics shortly after birth, which aids in the diagnosis of the condition.

Individuals who have Down syndrome may experience intellectual and developmental difficulties related to their cognitive ability. Despite the broad range of abilities, many people with Down syndrome lead happy, fulfilled lives when given the appropriate care and support. Early intervention therapies, such as speech and occupational therapy, can significantly enhance cognitive development and overall quality of life.

Additionally, there's a potential that those who have Down syndrome will have higher rates of thyroid issues, gastrointestinal problems, and cardiac anomalies. Regular medical check-ups and aggressive management of associated health issues are necessary to promote the well-being of individuals with Down syndrome.

Variations in Intensity

There can be notable variations in the severity of Down syndrome among individuals with the disorder while sharing a common genetic foundation. Numerous factors, such as the presence of additional medical conditions, the accessibility of early intervention services, and individual differences in cognitive ability, all have an impact on this diversity.

Some individuals with Down syndrome may require more help with everyday duties, while others may lead highly independent lives with very minor intellectual challenges. The variety of abilities and challenges emphasizes how important it is to provide tailored therapies to satisfy each person's unique needs.

To properly assist and educate, it is imperative to understand the disparities in severity. People with Down syndrome can benefit from individualized education plans, career development programs, and social integration activities to help them reach their full potential and participate in community life. Moreover, additional research into the factors influencing severity may help develop targeted interventions and therapies, enhancing the overall well-being and integration of individuals with Down syndrome.

CHAPTER THREE

EARLY RECOGNIZATION AND RESPONSE
Prenatal Testing and Counseling:

Prenatal testing and counseling play a major role in the early diagnosis and treatment of Down syndrome. Expectant parents can feel a range of emotions and concerns regarding the health of their unborn child. Prenatal testing provides a means of detecting genetic disorders like Down syndrome early in pregnancy. Both invasive procedures like amniocentesis and chorionic villus sampling (CVS) and non-invasive procedures like maternal serum screening and ultrasonography are commonly used in prenatal diagnosis for Down syndrome.

As part of a maternal serum screening technique, a pregnant woman's blood is tested for particular markers associated with Down syndrome. Conversely, ultrasound examinations can detect any anatomical irregularities that indicate the disease. During chorionic villus sampling and amniocentesis, respectively, a small sample of tissue or amniotic fluid is extracted for use in genetic analysis. Despite the remote possibility of side effects, these treatments offer a definitive diagnosis.

Counseling is an essential component of prenatal testing because it provides emotional support and helps parents deal with the emotional impact of a potential Down syndrome diagnosis. Genetic counselors play a crucial role in answering any questions and concerns that may arise, discussing choices, and providing information regarding test results. It is crucial to emphasize that prenatal testing is not necessary and that decisions on testing should be made after consulting medical specialists and taking into account one's own beliefs and circumstances.

In conclusion, prenatal testing and counseling are essential tools for educating potential parents about the health of their fetus. This proactive approach enables educated decision-making and prepares ahead of time for potential Down syndrome roadblocks.

Initial Symptoms and Recommendations:

It is crucial to identify signs and symptoms of Down syndrome early on to receive a diagnosis and begin treatment on time. While each individual with Down syndrome is unique, there are several physical and developmental characteristics that they all have that may raise concerns in an infant or young child.

Physical traits on the face such as almond-shaped eyes, flat nasal bridges, and projecting tongues are common in children with Down syndrome. They may also have reduced muscular tone and be lower in height. They may take longer than their peers to accomplish developmental milestones like walking, talking, or crawling. Another aspect of Down syndrome is cognitive challenges, such as learning disabilities and intellectual delays.

Parents and other caregivers must identify these warning signs and consult a physician for a comprehensive assessment. Early identification enables timely intervention that offers targeted therapy and specialized assistance to address specific developmental requirements. It is common practice to use occupational therapy, speech therapy, and physical therapy to enhance motor skills, communication capacity, and general cognitive development.

The importance of fostering a friendly and supportive environment cannot be overstated. Early intervention programs emphasize individualized educational techniques and therapies that significantly improve the overall well-being and potential of individuals with Down syndrome. With early detection and treatment, people with Down syndrome can realize their full potential and actively engage in many aspects of life.

The Importance of Early Intervention Programs

Early intervention programs are crucial for empowering individuals with Down syndrome and promoting their general development. These programs were initiated during the critical early years of life and are intended to address the unique demands and challenges associated with the disease. Early intervention employs a multidisciplinary strategy, with parents, educators, therapists, and medical professionals working together to optimize outcomes.

One of the primary goals of early intervention is to provide tailored support that addresses developmental deficits and promotes independence. Enhancing fine and gross motor skills, facilitating daily living activities, and improving coordination are the main objectives of occupational therapy. Through the resolution of communication issues, speech therapy improves communication skills in individuals with Down syndrome.

In addition, educational interventions are designed to recognize the benefits and drawbacks of the condition's cognitive aspects and accommodate a variety of learning styles.

Early intervention is beneficial not only for the individual with Down syndrome but also for their family. Parents and other caregivers are essential participants in these programs, receiving guidance on how to support their child's development at home. Early intervention promotes an inclusive society by assisting in the dismantling of barriers and misconceptions associated with Down syndrome.

Research consistently demonstrates that early intervention has a major positive impact on long-term outcomes and cognitive, social, and emotional development across time. Individuals with Down syndrome who receive early intervention are better able to acquire the skills necessary for an independent and self-assured life. These programs pay homage to the abilities and resilience of individuals with Down syndrome while highlighting the importance of an inclusive and encouraging environment from a young age.

CHAPTER FOUR

EXPERT ASSESSMENT AND SUPPORT
The Professional Advice of Genetic Counselors in Overcoming Down Syndrome

Genetic counselors are a vital component of the comprehensive plan for overcoming Down syndrome. Their primary responsibility is to provide families with up-to-date, reliable information regarding Down syndrome so they may better understand the disorder's genetic components. These professionals promote informed family planning choices by helping people comprehend the underlying genetic factors that cause Down syndrome.

Genetic counselors work with families both before and after the birth of a child with Down syndrome, answering questions and offering emotional support. They walk parents through the challenges of genetic testing and assist families in understanding the potential consequences and obtaining accurate findings. Genetic counselors use their expertise to assist affected families in seeing things more positively and intelligently, which significantly reduces uncertainties and anxieties about Down syndrome.

Additionally, genetic counselors play a crucial role in bridging the gap that exists between families and medical professionals by promoting effective communication. They act as advocates for individuals with Down syndrome, ensuring that their unique needs and issues are acknowledged and addressed by the broader healthcare system. Open communication and cooperation are key to the overall well-being of individuals with Down syndrome and their families, and genetic counselors play a crucial role in fostering these conditions.

A Pediatrician's Perspective on Overcoming Down Syndrome with Expert Guidance

Pediatricians' engagement is a crucial part of the multidisciplinary strategy to overcome Down syndrome. To provide timely, comprehensive medical care from the outset of a child's growth, pediatricians are essential. Early intervention is crucial since pediatricians are experts in recognizing developmental milestones and potential health issues associated with Down syndrome.

Pediatricians create individualized treatment plans in collaboration with other medical specialists that are tailored to each child with Down syndrome's unique needs. They monitor the physical and mental growth of the kid, identifying issues and implementing solutions as needed. In addition to providing families with advice on crucial subjects like nutrition, immunizations, and managing co-occurring medical conditions, pediatricians assess a child's overall health through routine examinations.

Furthermore, physicians play a crucial role in coordinating with educators and therapists to address the educational and developmental needs of children with Down syndrome. Because they recognize how important it is to assist each child in reaching their potential and becoming independent, they advocate warm and supportive learning settings.

Together with other professionals, pediatricians are essential in helping individuals with Down syndrome live better lives by providing ongoing medical treatment.

The Role of Specialized Therapists and Expert Counseling in Overcoming Down Syndrome

Involving specialist therapists is crucial to the comprehensive strategy for combating Down syndrome. These medical professionals, which include speech, occupational, and physical therapists, assist individuals with Down syndrome in their entire development and well-being.

Speech therapists focus on improving communication skills, addressing speech problems, and promoting language development. Through tailored interventions, they support individuals in expressing themselves appropriately, fostering social interaction and self-assurance. By fostering the growth of fine motor skills, sensory integration, and daily living tasks, occupational therapists hope to foster independence and autonomy in their patients.

Physical therapists are important when it comes to treating motor issues, promoting physical fitness, and enhancing overall mobility. Their programs aim to enable persons with Down syndrome to participate actively in a range of physical activities through enhanced muscle strength, balance, and coordination. By meeting their unique needs, specialized therapists assist individuals with Down syndrome in developing cognitively and physically, allowing them to lead fulfilling lives.

In summary, the collaborative efforts of medical professionals, licensed therapists, and genetic counselors yield a comprehensive and supportive basis for conquering Down syndrome. By their unique responsibilities, these professionals help individuals with Down syndrome succeed and have fulfilling lives. They also give their families the knowledge and resources they need to live a happy, inclusive life.

CHAPTER FIVE

METHODS OF INSTRUCTION
Tailoring Educational Plans to Individual Students:

Lesson plans that are specifically designed are necessary to satisfy the educational demands of individuals with Down syndrome. To create a customized education for every student, it is essential to recognize their unique abilities, challenges, and learning styles. Since there is a wide range of developmental profiles and talents associated with Down syndrome, there is no one-size-fits-all solution.

To understand the cognitive and socioemotional components of every kid, teachers should conduct thorough assessments. Finding one's strengths—such as oral communication, visual learning, or memory—is necessary for this. Whether it is with language development, athletic abilities, or social interaction, identifying the areas that require further support is essential.

Setting realistic, reachable goals that include each student's abilities is necessary to create learning programs that are customized to meet their needs. Hard tasks can be broken down into smaller, more manageable steps so that one can advance gradually and build confidence along the way. Specialized teaching methods, such as multimodal approaches and visual aids, may be employed to enhance the learning process. Regular assessments and adjustments ensure that the learning plan remains flexible and adaptable to each student's unique needs.

The establishment of a friendly and inclusive learning environment is equally crucial. The effectiveness of personalized lesson plans is increased when parents, caregivers, and educators work together as a team. Clear channels of communication facilitate the exchange of ideas and provide a thorough approach to each person's education. Encouraging people with Down syndrome to realize their full potential and participate actively in the educational process is the ultimate goal.

Inclusive Education Models:

The use of inclusive education models becomes crucial in the educational battle against Down syndrome. More than merely being physically present in a typical classroom, inclusion for those with Down syndrome emphasizes social integration, active participation, and a sense of belonging.

A key element of inclusive education is the creation of a welcoming school environment. Fostering acceptance, empathy, and understanding between teachers and students is part of this. Schools should employ peer support networks, awareness campaigns, and anti-bullying programs to promote an inclusive culture that celebrates diversity.

Customizing the curriculum is another crucial component of inclusive education. It involves modifying educational materials, tactics, and evaluation approaches to meet a variety of learning demands. This may mean providing additional time for understanding, incorporating practical exercises, and using visual aids for those with Down syndrome. Differentiated education makes it possible for every student, regardless of ability, to access and engage with the material efficiently.

Collaboration between special education professionals, support staff, and teachers is necessary for inclusive education strategies. Regular meetings to discuss professional development, share strategies, and address roadblocks promote a cohesive and effective approach. Professional development programs that focus on understanding and supporting the unique needs of individuals with Down syndrome serve to reinforce the inclusive education framework.

Academic success is not the only factor that matters in inclusive education; social skills and emotional stability are equally crucial. People with Down syndrome can interact with their peers through extracurricular activities, social events, and inclusive playgrounds to break down barriers and foster a sense of community.

Technology for Education Developed with Down Syndrome in Mind:

The integration of educational technology holds great potential to enhance the academic performance of people with Down syndrome. Well-designed and customized digital solutions can address specific cognitive challenges associated with Down syndrome, provide tailored education, and enhance communication skills.

One notable area of the application of educational technology is the realm of assistive communication devices. Augmentative and alternative communication (AAC) devices can be very beneficial for people with Down syndrome when it comes to expressive language. These instruments, which help individuals communicate effectively, can range in complexity from graphic communication boards to speech-generating devices.

Interactive educational software and apps made with the universal learning design (UDL) principles can support a wide range of learning methods and ability levels. These programs often incorporate multimedia elements, interactive exercises, and flexible features that allow for personalized progress. Apps that prioritize visual learning and interactive storytelling, for instance, may be especially beneficial for those who have Down syndrome.

Furthermore, virtual reality (VR) and augmented reality (AR) technologies offer immersive learning experiences. These technologies can simulate real-world scenarios in virtual environments, which could make learning more engaging and beneficial. People with Down syndrome, who might benefit from practical learning through hands-on activities, might have a unique and meaningful educational experience with these tools.

In the digital age, increasing access to educational opportunities requires the use of online platforms and resources. Web-based courses, video tutorials, and interactive learning platforms provide persons with Down syndrome with access to educational content in a format that suits their learning preferences and at their own pace. These platforms can be enhanced with ongoing support from educators and caregivers to ensure a thorough educational experience.

To summarize, the integration of educational technology for people with Down syndrome requires a thoughtful and all-encompassing approach. It means not only selecting the right materials but also providing the guidance and support needed to maximize the educational potential of technology for individuals with Down syndrome.

CHAPTER SIX

MEDICAL ADMINISTRATION
Medical Concerns and Frequently Scheduled Exams:

A genetic disorder called Down syndrome is brought on by an extra copy of chromosome 21. People who have this illness could have particular difficulties that call for close medical supervision. It needs professional assistance to navigate the medical considerations associated with Down syndrome. Regular check-ups are crucial for monitoring an individual's overall health and for swiftly treating any emerging problems.

Medical considerations have a great deal of interest in developmental assessments. Early intervention is crucial to give the proper kind of support for cognitive and physical development. Regular evaluations carried out by doctors and developmental specialists allow for the early identification of developmental milestones and delays. Customized actions that can enhance an individual's quality of life and enable them to realize their full potential are made possible by these evaluations.

In addition to cognitive delays, heart abnormalities, thyroid issues, and digestive problems are common health issues experienced by individuals with Down syndrome. With the aid of professional supervision, these illnesses can be controlled by targeted screenings and therapy. Cardiologists may do routine cardiac testing to find and treat any anomalies in the heart, whereas endocrinologists monitor thyroid function to prevent problems related to it. These medical issues emphasize the importance of a multidisciplinary approach to healthcare management, which entails multiple professionals collaborating to provide comprehensive and customized care.

Professional guidance may also be beneficial for the individual with Down syndrome's family and caregivers. Through early intervention strategies, preventive measures, and education about potential health hazards, families are empowered to take an active role in their loved one's care. The collaborative approach fosters a supportive environment that enhances the overall quality of life for individuals with Down syndrome.

Nutrition and Well-Being:

When it comes to managing their overall healthcare, wellness, and nutrition are extremely important for people with Down syndrome. Expert advice in these areas aims to optimize physical health, cognitive function, and overall quality of life. A complete approach that addresses the unique requirements of individuals with Down syndrome includes tailored exercise routines, specific dietary considerations, and ongoing wellness support.

One of the most crucial nutritional considerations for individuals with Down syndrome is addressing the likelihood of obesity. Their genetic make-up, slow metabolism, and decreased muscle tone can predispose individuals to weight-related issues. A diet plan that balances physical activity with calorie consumption to support good weight management should be created under the guidance of an expert. Dietitians work closely with their clients' families to create long-term health-promoting eating habits.

In addition to dietary considerations, expert counsel emphasizes the importance of regular exercise. Exercise helps people regulate their weight and enhances their cardiovascular health, muscular tone, and coordination. Exercise programs that are customized to the unique physical requirements of individuals with Down syndrome are crucial for promoting an active and healthy way of life.

Mental health concerns are included in the support for wellness. Along with social challenges, people with Down syndrome may also struggle with mental health conditions including anxiety or depression. Expert advice includes strategies for promoting resilience, mental health, and social inclusion. Psychologists and counselors play a crucial role in advancing a holistic view of wellness by providing Down syndrome individuals and their families with information and assistance.

Taking Care of Typical Medical Issues:

Down syndrome is associated with several common health issues, which require specialized care and informed guidance for effective management. For individuals with Down syndrome, proactive approaches such as early discovery, intervention, and ongoing monitoring are required to address these health issues and ensure the best potential outcomes.

Regular cardiovascular assessments are crucial to the treatment of Down syndrome because the condition is frequently associated with cardiac problems in those who have it. Under the supervision of a specialist, specialized cardiac screenings are carried out to find congenital heart defects and other cardiovascular conditions. Early intervention, which is typically accomplished by surgical procedures or medical care, can significantly improve long-term cardiac outcomes.

Thyroid issues are another common medical complication among individuals with Down syndrome. Thyroid function, particularly thyroid hormone levels, needs to be routinely examined for early detection and treatment. To prevent difficulties and advance overall health, endocrinologists work closely with patients and their medical teams to ensure that thyroid-related issues are promptly addressed.

Gastrointestinal (GI) conditions including celiac disease and digestive issues are major concerns for those with Down syndrome. Expert advice for GI issues includes dietary modifications, nutritional support, and routine monitoring to increase digestive health and controlling symptoms. Collaboration between gastroenterologists, dietitians, and other healthcare professionals is necessary to implement personalized treatments that appropriately address these common health issues.

Professional guidance covers more than just these specific health concerns; it also involves a thorough plan for handling the treatment of patients with Down syndrome. This covers comprehensive dental care, individualized immunizations, and eye and hearing tests.

Several professionals working together to coordinate care provide a thorough and personalized approach to treating common health issues in individuals with Down syndrome.

In conclusion, expert help is essential for handling medical concerns, wellness and nutrition, and common health issues associated with Down syndrome. Healthcare professionals from multiple specializations work together in a multidisciplinary approach to provide persons with Down syndrome with a comprehensive and customized treatment plan that maximizes their potential and well-being. People with Down syndrome can lead happy, healthy lives with the support of a network of experts who are dedicated to fulfilling their unique needs. This network includes proactive medical treatment, dietary assistance, and targeted interventions.

CHAPTER SEVEN

PSYCHOSOCIAL GROWTH
How Emotional Intelligence Can Be Developed

The psychosocial development of individuals with Down syndrome depends on their ability to develop emotional intelligence. Emotional intelligence includes the capacity to recognize, understand, and control one's own emotions as well as empathy for others. People with Down syndrome can benefit greatly from the development of emotional intelligence in both their social interactions and overall well-being.

Experts often oversee the use of specialized therapies that prioritize emotional expression, management, and comprehension to develop emotional intelligence in individuals with Down syndrome. These solutions may include specialized therapy like emotional coaching, which teaches people how to identify and communicate their feelings. Emotional intelligence can also be greatly aided by play therapy and other activities that heighten emotional awareness, such as painting.

Establishing a safe space that encourages emotional expression without passing judgment is a responsibility for caregivers and professionals. Recognizing and validating their emotions helps people with Down syndrome become more emotionally intelligent. People can also learn coping strategies and stress management techniques under the supervision of professionals, which will help them navigate their emotional landscapes with resilience.

Gaining Social Competencies

People with Down syndrome need to learn social skills to grow psychosocially. It needs professional help to develop strategies that encourage fruitful social encounters and long-lasting friendships. The phrase "social skills" encompasses a wide range of abilities, including collaboration, communication, and the ability to read social cues. These skills are necessary for engaging in a range of social situations.

For individuals with Down syndrome, specific programs frequently aim to build effective communication skills. Specialists regularly employ social skills instruction, speech therapy, and augmentative and alternative communication (AAC) methods.

These therapies are made to specifically address the needs of individuals with Down syndrome, emphasizing both their strengths and possible challenges.

Participating in community events and being exposed to social surroundings can also significantly contribute to the development of social skills. In collaboration with educational institutions, neighborhood associations, and support groups, inclusive settings can be developed where individuals with Down syndrome can refine and enhance their social skills under the direction of professionals. These programs are essential for encouraging social integration and independence.

Community And Family Support

The community's and family's support are crucial pillars in the psychological development of individuals with Down syndrome. Expert counsel emphasizes how important it is to build a support system outside of one's immediate family. This network of friends, educators, health professionals, and community groups works together to enhance the overall quality of life for those with Down syndrome.

Professional support in the family often involves providing resources and information to help family members comprehend Down syndrome. This category may include educational, therapeutic, and support group programs that offer a space for sharing experiences and coping techniques. Experts also stress the need to foster a warm, supportive family environment that upholds each member's autonomy and sense of value.

To promote tolerance and diversity in the greater community, professionals collaborate with businesses, educational institutions, and recreational groups. This can mean advocating for inclusive laws and training educators and employers on how to effectively support individuals with Down syndrome. Expert counsel recognizes the importance of a supportive community in lowering stigma and ensuring that individuals with Down syndrome can lead fulfilling lives.

CHAPTER EIGHT

THERAPEUTIC APPROACHES
Speech-language pathology in Down syndrome patients:

Disabilities with speech and language are among the most common problems that people with Down syndrome encounter. Speech-language therapy, or SLT, is crucial for addressing these issues and promoting effective communication methods. Part of the professional advice in this therapeutic approach includes a comprehensive assessment of the patient's speech and language abilities, taking into consideration their unique strengths and limits.

Speech-language pathologists work closely with individuals with Down syndrome to enhance their articulation, vocabulary expansion, and expressive language. These experts understand that individuals with Down syndrome have a wide variety of speech and language abilities, and they tailor interventions to each person's specific needs.

A key element of speech therapy is early intervention, which starts as soon as feasible to maximize language development. Therapists use augmentative and alternative communication, or AAC, as one strategy to support individuals with Down syndrome in expressing themselves. In SLT, professional supervision also entails collaborating with educators, caregivers, and other experts to create a thorough plan for enhancing communication.

Additionally, a key element of speech therapy is social communication skills. Counselors assist individuals with Down syndrome in establishing strong bonds and relationships as well as navigating social settings. With an emphasis on functional communication and individual interests, expert-guided speech and language therapy can significantly improve the overall quality of life for people with Down syndrome.

Occupational treatment for people with Down syndrome:

Occupational therapy (OT) is a successful therapeutic approach that focuses on enhancing daily living skills and encouraging independence for individuals with Down syndrome. In occupational therapy, professional supervision involves a comprehensive assessment of the patient's strengths, weaknesses, and specific needs for activities of daily living (ADLs).

Occupational therapists develop tailored interventions focusing on fine and gross motor skills, self-care skills, and sensory processing in partnership with families and individuals with Down syndrome. For example, fine motor skills can be targeted with handwriting practice, and gross motor skills can be addressed with play and exercise.

Expert-led occupational therapy also considers sensory processing problems, which are commonly associated with Down syndrome. Therapists use sensory integration strategies to help people better control and understand sensory information. Clients are better able to focus, pay attention, and feel better all over as a result. Using adaptive methods and technologies to increase independence with daily tasks could also be suggested.

In addition to individual sessions, occupational therapy often includes integrating therapeutic activities into a patient's home, school, and community contexts. Collaboration is emphasized heavily in expert guidance, with teachers and caregivers needing to be equipped with the knowledge and skills necessary to appropriately support the client's occupational therapy goals.

Physical Therapy And Exercise In The Context Of Down Syndrome:

Physical therapy and exercise are essential components of a comprehensive therapeutic approach for individuals with Down syndrome. For professional help in this area, a thorough assessment of the individual's motor abilities, musculoskeletal development, and physical capacities is required. The goals are to improve overall health, improve motor coordination, and increase physical fitness.

Physical therapists help individuals with Down syndrome get past specific motor challenges like weak muscles, loose joints, and balance issues. Customized exercise plans aim to address these areas with a focus on strength training, flexibility, and coordination. Physical therapy under the supervision of experts recognizes the importance of tailoring treatments to each patient's unique needs and abilities.

In addition to treating specific motor impairments, physical therapy is crucial for preventing and controlling secondary health issues that may arise in individuals with Down syndrome. These include encouraging an active lifestyle, combating obesity, and improving cardiovascular health.

In contexts other than the clinic, physical therapists collaborate with educators, caregivers, and other medical specialists. Therapists educate their patients on the importance of regular exercise, how to follow at-home fitness plans, and how to promote an active and healthy lifestyle. By integrating physical therapy into their daily routine, expert-guided therapies assist persons with Down syndrome to live better lives overall and in terms of their physical health.

CHAPTER NINE

INVESTIGATIONS AND NOVELTIES
Recent Advances in the Research on Down Syndrome:

In the past few years, research on Down syndrome (DS) has advanced significantly, shedding light on the complex genetic and physiological aspects of this condition. One significant achievement is the identification of specific genes and genetic pathways linked to DS. Modern genomic technology has been used by researchers to sort through the complex gene-to-gene interactions on chromosome 21, the source of the extra copy in DS patients. This increased comprehension has opened the door for certain treatment interventions in addition to offering crucial insights into the molecular mechanisms underlying DS.

Moreover, advances in neuroimaging methods have made it possible for researchers to study the functional and structural components of the brain in people with Down syndrome. Different patterns of brain growth and connectivity have been shown by these studies, which has advanced our understanding of the neurological and cognitive characteristics associated with Down syndrome. These developments are essential for creating tailored interventions that target the unique problems that people with Down syndrome encounter at different stages of their lives.

Along with developments in neuroscience and genetics, recent studies have explored the role of epigenetic modifications in Down syndrome. It has been shown that epigenetic processes—which alter gene expression without changing the underlying DNA sequence—have a significant impact on the development of traits associated with Down syndrome. Comprehending these epigenetic modifications presents novel prospects for treatment strategies that endeavor to regulate gene expression to mitigate the effects of Down syndrome on cognitive and physical maturation.

Improvements in early diagnosis and intervention strategies have also resulted from collaborations between researchers and medical professionals. Early identification of DS indicators increases the likelihood of positive outcomes by enabling timely and tailored therapy. Together, these developments represent a paradigm shift in DS research, moving the field away from a symptomatic approach and toward a more focused and nuanced understanding of the illness.

Potential Medicines and Procedures:

Promising cures and treatments have emerged in the battle against Down syndrome, giving those with the condition and their families greater hope. One important field of study is the use of pharmaceuticals to target particular genetic pathways linked to Down syndrome. The cognitive and developmental issues linked to DS may be resolved by tiny molecules and drugs that try to change gene expression or boost neuroplasticity.

There are now effective ways to improve the quality of life for people with DS, including behavioral and cognitive therapy. Specialized educational plans and therapeutic interventions, like occupational and speech therapy, have demonstrated remarkable effectiveness in treating issues related to motor skills and communication. The development of independence and improvement of general well-being can be achieved by early and regular access to these therapies.

Moreover, the field of regenerative medicine has demonstrated potential in producing new DS treatments. Particularly, stem cell therapies can replace or repair damaged tissues and cells, addressing DS's physical and cognitive aspects. These regenerative approaches, albeit still in the early stages of development, mark a significant advancement toward more all-encompassing and revolutionary treatments for individuals with Down syndrome.

Apart from these therapeutic approaches, advancements in assistive technologies have been significant in enabling people with Down syndrome. Technological advancements like communication devices, mobility aids, and adaptive technologies have significantly improved accessibility and inclusion, allowing people with Down syndrome to participate more completely in different aspects of life.

Prospects for Further Research on Down Syndrome:

The direction of research on Down syndrome is expected to change shortly, with a focus on individualized and precise care. With the development of genomic medicine, personalized genetic profiles can now be identified, allowing for the development of individualized medicines based on the unique genetic makeup of patients with DS. This tactic can reduce side effects and increase treatment outcomes.

Furthermore, future research endeavors are anticipated to be propelled by a shift toward multidisciplinary collaboration. A thorough understanding of DS will be possible through the integration of research from genetics, neuroscience, psychology, and other pertinent domains. This will also facilitate the development of all-encompassing remedies that tackle the myriad problems linked to the illness. Researcher, healthcare professional, and advocacy group collaboration will be essential to creating a more accepting and encouraging atmosphere for people with Down syndrome.

Technological developments, especially in the areas of artificial intelligence and machine learning, are probably going to be crucial in the analysis of large datasets and the discovery of complex patterns associated with data science. These instruments could expedite the rate of discovery and enhance our comprehension of the intricate interactions of genetic, environmental, and epigenetic factors in developmental disorders.

Moreover, future studies are probably going to find more value in emphasizing early intervention and preventative measures. The possibility of enhancing long-term results for individuals with Down syndrome exists through the identification of biomarkers and early indicators of DS risk and the development of customized therapeutics throughout pivotal stages of the disease's development.

The ethical ramifications of new scientific discoveries and technological advancements will likewise gain more attention as science advances. The responsible development and application of future medications and treatments for Down syndrome will depend heavily on striking a balance between the potential advantages of scientific advancement and ethical considerations, such as concerns about consent, privacy, and social impact.

CHAPTER TEN

PARENTAL COUNSELING AND SUPPORT
Developing Parents' Advocacy Skills:

Having parents become activists is essential to combating Down syndrome with knowledgeable assistance. Parents have a significant influence on the opportunities and quality of life available to their children with Down syndrome, and they also play a vital part in their lives.

Providing parents with comprehensive information about Down syndrome, including its medical characteristics, educational implications, and societal viewpoints, is essential to empowering them. A parent with knowledge can more effectively navigate the challenges associated with raising a child with Down syndrome.

Professional supervision includes equipping parents with the knowledge and skills necessary to successfully navigate the healthcare system, comprehend treatment approaches, and obtain educational materials tailored to their child's specific needs. Experts in special education, medicine, genetic counseling, and other fields can provide information on the most recent developments in therapy, pedagogy, and research. By having access to this information, parents may make well-informed decisions regarding the care of their children and can participate actively in the decision-making process.

Creating a feeling of camaraderie among parents of kids with Down syndrome is also essential. Bringing together parents who have similar experiences creates a support system that extends beyond expert advice. Peer support helps parents learn from each other and share strategies for conquering challenges by providing emotional resilience and useful insights. Proficient parents, knowledgeable about both professional advice and the combined power of life experiences, grow into outstanding advocates for their kids, promoting diversity and shattering social barriers.

Resources and Support Systems:

Overcoming Down syndrome with professional assistance requires creating strong support networks and making resources easily accessible. The benefits of a multidisciplinary approach involving educators, healthcare providers, and community organizations are enormous for individuals with Down syndrome. Support networks must be all-encompassing, incorporating social, educational, and medical components to meet the various requirements that people with Down syndrome have throughout their lives.

Pediatricians, genetic counselors, and other specialists who can guide early treatments, managing healthcare, and potential co-occurring diseases should collaborate to form medical support networks. Teachers with expertise in inclusive classrooms, individualized education plans (IEPs), and special education methodologies should be part of educational support networks.

Furthermore, enhancing cooperation between parents and schools strengthens the whole support system, guaranteeing that the educational needs of people with Down syndrome are effectively satisfied.

In addition to the fields of medicine and education, social support networks play a critical role in promoting social acceptance and inclusion. Social clubs, advocacy groups, and community organizations that specifically serve people with Down syndrome can foster a feeling of community and help with social skill development. It is equally important to dispel stigmas and foster an inclusive attitude in the larger community so that people with Down syndrome can live fulfilling lives.

Accessible resources are essential for empowering parents and individuals with Down syndrome. These resources include informational materials, online communities, and neighborhood community centers. These resources should be tailored to the unique issues and possibilities related to Down syndrome, providing support with independent living, independent healthcare, education, and careers.

Legal Rights and Defenses:

A thorough understanding of and advocacy for the legal rights and safeguards afforded to individuals with Down syndrome and their families is necessary to defeat the condition with the help of experts. To guarantee that people with Down syndrome have equal access to opportunities, services, and protection from discrimination, legal frameworks are essential.

Promoting inclusive education policies is a crucial component. Laws should ensure that students with Down syndrome receive an education appropriate to their particular needs, promoting inclusive classrooms and providing access to specialized support services. This involves creating and carrying out individualized education plans (IEPs) that cater to the unique learning needs of every student.

Legal rights also have to cover healthcare. The goal of advocacy efforts should be to ensure that everyone has equal access to high-quality healthcare services. This involves making certain that healthcare professionals are suitably qualified to provide suitable care for people with Down syndrome and that insurance covers the required therapies, interventions, and treatments.

The prevention of discrimination in the workplace is another important issue. The rights of individuals with Down syndrome in the workplace should be safeguarded by legislative frameworks, which should provide them with equal opportunity, protection from discrimination, and reasonable accommodations. Campaigns to raise awareness and encourage workplace diversity can contribute to the development of work cultures that support the professional achievement of individuals with Down syndrome.

In addition, legal frameworks ought to address broader societal issues including housing, transportation, and community inclusion. This means advocating for accessible public spaces, accessible transit, and housing options that consider the unique needs of individuals with Down syndrome.

In conclusion, conquering Down syndrome under the guidance of a professional requires fighting for legal rights and safeguards and being aware of them. Individuals with Down syndrome can lead fulfilling lives with equal rights and protections, provided that society makes sure laws are comprehensive and inclusive.

CHAPTER ELEVEN

ACCOMPLISHMENTS AND INSPIRATION
Qualities of Successful Down Syndrome Individuals

Numerous successes in the field of conquering Down syndrome under professional supervision show how resilient and capable individuals with the condition may be. One such inspiring tale is that of Alex, who, with the assistance of dedicated professionals, has developed into a useful member of society. Alex was diagnosed at an early age, and his narrative serves as an example of how expert guidance may have a transformative effect. Alex has succeeded in many areas of life after overcoming developmental challenges and getting specialist therapies like occupational therapy, speech therapy, and educational help.

Beyond reaching his objectives, Alex has made a lasting contribution to education. Despite outdated stereotypes, individuals with Down syndrome can achieve academic success with the right support. By pursuing more education and completing high school under the guidance of qualified teachers in welcoming classrooms, Alex dismantled barriers. His academic success serves as proof of the benefits of tailored instruction and the potential that every person, regardless of genetic makeup, possesses.

Achievements in sports and the workforce serve as further evidence of the triumph over Down syndrome. Sarah's narrative challenges preconceived notions about physical strength. Sarah is a gifted athlete. Sarah played competitive sports and did well under the direction of coaches and specialized training regimens, proving that having Down syndrome does not stop someone from reaching their athletic ambitions. A person with Down syndrome has a wide range of skills and abilities, which are demonstrated by their success in the job, whether in the arts or business. People are not only overcoming challenges but also significantly improving a wide range of professional disciplines under the guidance of pros.

These stories demonstrate how a person with Down syndrome can have a happy and fulfilling life if they receive the appropriate support. These success stories are a source of inspiration for individuals going through similar struggles because they demonstrate the value of early intervention, individualized support, and accepting environments.

Achievements in Athletics, Education, and Professions:

With expert help, people with Down syndrome can overcome the condition and achieve remarkable success in a range of areas, including work, sports, and education. Education-wise, new techniques and tailored interventions have allowed individuals with Down syndrome to participate in mainstream school settings and achieve academic success. With the help of specialized curricula, inclusive education tactics, and the steadfast guidance of dedicated teachers, children such as Emily have overcome insurmountable obstacles to achieve previously unthinkable academic goals.

In other sports-related success stories, individuals with Down syndrome have not only embraced physical activity but also excelled in competitive environments. Coaches and sports organizations have been key actors in developing flexible training programs that encourage participation and acknowledge successes. The story of Michael, a young swimmer with Down syndrome, shows how professional sports coaching can develop latent potential while promoting physical well-being and a sense of accomplishment.

Furthermore, a paradigm change is occurring in the professional environment as an increasing number of individuals with Down syndrome pursue successful careers. The narrative of Jessica, a graphic artist, debunks stereotypes regarding the employability of individuals with Down syndrome. Through job accommodations, vocational training, and mentoring programs, Jessica not only found a rewarding job but also developed into a proponent of the inclusion of people with disabilities in a range of professions.

These successes in the classroom, on the field, and in the workforce demonstrate how transformative professional mentoring can be. By recognizing and leveraging individual abilities, implementing inclusive practices, and offering ongoing support, society can create opportunities for the meaningful and prosperous involvement of people with Down syndrome in various fields.

Respecting Diversity and Eradicating Preconceptions:

Beyond individual accomplishments, overcoming Down syndrome with expert help entails embracing diversity and dispelling the long-held misconceptions about this inherited condition. Each success story dispels misconceptions and advances an inclusive society by showcasing the wide variety of talents and proficiencies among people with Down syndrome.

One beautiful aspect of this celebration of variety is the flourishing artistic expression of individuals with Down syndrome. People like Liam can express their unique qualities and personalities through a range of artistic genres, including visual and performing arts.

People with Down syndrome can challenge social conventions and contribute to culture through art therapy, which becomes a powerful instrument for self-expression and personal development when paired with professional supervision.

Eliminating preconceptions also extends to the social realm, where ties to the community and community involvement are essential. The story of Olivia, who has developed close relationships in her community, debunks the misconception that individuals with Down syndrome could find it challenging to socialize. Olivia has become a voice for acceptance and understanding in addition to creating lifelong connections with the aid of community projects and social inclusion initiatives.

In conclusion, both the celebration of diversity and the demolition of stereotypes are essential components of the fight against Down syndrome. Expert guidance transcends personal achievements to modify societal perceptions and cultivate an environment that values the unique characteristics of individuals with Down syndrome.